You inspire me to be better!
Thank you for leading me on
this wild ride of a doctorate!
D

Breast Cancer Mardi Gras

*Surviving the Emotional Hurricane
and Showing My Boobs to Strangers*

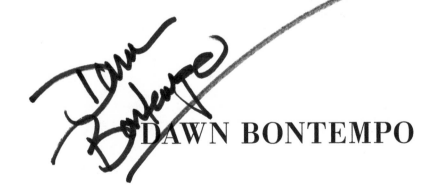

DAWN BONTEMPO

authorHOUSE®

You inspire me to be better!
Thank you for leading me on
this wild ride of a doctorate!

AuthorHouse™
1663 Liberty Drive
Bloomington, IN 47403
www.authorhouse.com
Phone: 1-800-839-8640

Published by AuthorHouse 07/23/13

ISBN: 978-1-4918-0315-8 (sc)
ISBN: 978-1-4918-0316-5 (hc)
ISBN: 978-1-4918-0399-8 (e)

Library of Congress Control Number: 2013913347

Any people depicted in stock imagery provided by Thinkstock are models,
and such images are being used for illustrative purposes only.
Certain stock imagery © Thinkstock.

This book is printed on acid-free paper.

Because of the dynamic nature of the Internet, any web addresses or links contained in
this book may have changed since publication and may no longer be valid. The views
expressed in this work are solely those of the author and do not necessarily reflect the
views of the publisher, and the publisher hereby disclaims any responsibility for them.

To Dori:

You are exceedingly awesome, tremendously funny, and the best sister ever. Thank you for always picking up the phone to listen to my craziness, talking me off the ledge when necessary, and, of course, capturing our conversations! I continue to learn from you every day.

To Felix:

You are extremely supportive and exceptionally encouraging. Thank you for being my playmate in life. Love always.

To Mom and Dad:

You instilled in me the ability to laugh when times get tough. Thank you for a childhood filled with fun and laughter and with enough life lessons to make me who I am today. It is an honor to call you Mom and Dad.

To my family and friends:

You are the reason I wrote this book. The support, assistance, and love I received during this journey propelled me to keep fighting and keep writing. Thank you. I am forever grateful.

Table of Contents

Introduction

Sister: "How do you feel?"

Me: "It's like I have the worst hangover ever with the added suffering of the flu. I'm nauseous; I ache all over; I feel miserable. I slept on my bathroom floor. It's horrible. [Insert more awful stuff.] So what's new with you?"

Sister: "Ummmmm ... I have a zit ..."

Me: (silence) ... (and then I burst out laughing!)

IF YOU ARE READING this book, you are probably either fighting your own cancer battle or have a friend who is fighting. Here are a few things you should know about me.

- I am not the kind of person who sits back and waits for life to happen to me. I want *action*, and I want it now!
- I am sarcastic and usually able to find something funny about most situations.
- I am blessed to have supportive family and friends, including a sister who kept me laughing through the entire ordeal.
- I was forty-one years old when I was diagnosed with breast cancer, which made me mad as hell.

When I was diagnosed, I laughed. I cried. I drank wine. I bought new underwear (we'll get to that). I laughed some more. Breast cancer is a serious topic. However, for me to mentally get through this journey, I had to poke fun at some of the absurdities along the way, such as the number of doctors and nurses playing with my boobs, squishing my boobs, poking my boobs, positioning my boobs, and—who could forget?—taking photos of my boobs. Yes, there were boob photos! Lots and lots of boob photos! And although I was horrified, a tiny voice inside my head wondered if I should request copies for my fiancé.

Boob photos were just the beginning. There was the absurdity of baring my butt to doctors after my chemo side effects produced an awesome abscess there. Oh yes, there was a butt abscess. I didn't request photos.

This book is chaptered as a series of *actions*. The actions are meant as suggestions, as everyone's fight will be different, but my hope is that you will gather information from my successes and learn from those things I could have done better. The start of each chapter is a conversation between my sister and me. My sister took her job of number one cheerleader and therapist very seriously. She offered advice, council, and humor on a daily basis. I wrap up each chapter with unsolicited advice based on my experience going through this process.

I hope you find my breast cancer story educational and humorous with just the right amount of sarcasm added in for fun. I give you my real life experience and descriptions, even of those things that were not so pleasant. Good luck with your battle and keep laughing!

Part 1

The Diagnosis–How I Found Out I Had Breast Cancer

C ANCER ... CANCER? CANCER!

I found out I had breast cancer at 2:00 p.m. on Friday, October 12, but my story began on Saturday, September 29.

September 29 was my twin nephews' fourth birthday party, and I was driving to Pennsylvania to celebrate. All day I felt a sharp, shooting pain in my left breast. If you have done any research, pain is not an indication of breast cancer. So, as I am prone to do, I ignored it. Within twenty-four hours, no more pain. Yippee! I had nothing to worry about anymore.

Within a few days, I noticed an indentation (I would later find out this is referred to as dimpling). I was pretty sure the indentation had not been on my breast the day before ... and neither had the lump that was now present. I thought, *This sucks*, and then I ignored it!

I traveled back to Pennsylvania to spend the following weekend at Penn State with my sister and her family. We attended the Penn State football game, and while traveling to and from the game, I told my sister about my pain and the indentation. She politely—as in,

Dawn Bontempo

"I will kick your ass if you don't"—asked me to see a doctor when I returned to Virginia. I promised that I would. I'm kind of afraid of my sister.

On Tuesday, October 9, I made an appointment with my primary care clinician. She checked me out and recommended a mammogram that day. (Clue number one that I should have paid attention to – the clinician sent me for a mammogram the same day as my appointment!)

The mammogram was scheduled for 3:00 p.m. My last mammogram had only been eighteen months before, so I wasn't too worried. My breasts were pressed between two plates until I thought I would faint, and then I was sent back to the waiting area. The tech came back in a few minutes and said the radiologist wanted more pictures. So I was jammed back into the machine and sent back to the waiting area. The tech came back in a few more minutes and said the radiologist recommended an ultrasound. So I was escorted to another room for the ultrasound. During the ultrasound, the tech spent a lot of time in my armpit. When I asked why, she said she was looking at the lymph nodes. (Clue number two that I should have paid attention to—the tech spent more time in the ultrasound looking at lymph nodes than looking at my breast.)

The tech left to talk to the radiologist. The radiologist joined the party and recommended a biopsy. She had already spoken with my primary care clinician, and they recommended the biopsy now. *(Now?)* So they wheeled in a cart and performed a needle biopsy. For the record, it *hurt!* (Clue number three that I should have paid attention to—the health care system was so efficient that I had an appointment, a mammogram, an ultrasound, and a biopsy in the same day!)

I went home and tried to ignore these clues. I was pretty successful until Friday, October 12, at 2:00 p.m., when the radiologist called my office. She did not say, "You have cancer." She called and said,

2

"The test results were positive." Intellectually, I understood what that meant. But *positive* means "good," doesn't it? In my world, it does. But in this situation, *positive* meant that I had breast cancer.

I had "moderately differentiated, infiltrating ductal carcinoma." It took a lot of Internet searches to figure out what that meant, but at that moment, the only thing I knew was that I had cancer. Now what?

Chapter 1

Action–Get Your Peeps Lined Up

Me: "How do I tell people I have cancer?"

Sister: "What are you thinking?"

Me: "I'm thinking about a Facebook post."

Sister: (silence) "Well. That's one way."

Me: "Do you have a better idea?"

Sister: "Not really."

Me: "Well, here goes. I'm pushing 'post' for my 'I have cancer' Facebook post."

Sister: "You didn't really want my advice, did you? What if I'd had a better idea?"

Me: "I wouldn't have hit 'post'!"

THERE'S NOTHING LIKE A cancer diagnosis to mobilize your friends! You will need help! You might as well start getting the help lined up from the very beginning.

My first big question was: "How do I tell folks?" I had no idea what to say. After a lot of trial and error, I realized folks had no idea what to say to me either. Once I figured this out, I was very open about my diagnosis and my fight. I also tried to put folks at ease by explaining I knew they didn't know what to say, but neither did I, and together we'd figure it out. I also smiled a lot and told funny, absurd stories about what I was going through; this again put folks at ease. Cancer is serious business, but I couldn't be serious all the time—it was way too exhausting!

I was diagnosed at 2:00 p.m. on a Friday afternoon while sitting at my desk in my office. I hung up with the radiologist and immediately called my sister. My sister is a caring, generous, and loving person—who also believes in sarcasm and action. After crying for a few minutes with her, I had a "real" dilemma to solve. I had closed the door to my office when the radiologist called. In order for me to leave, I had to walk by a whole lot of folks.

So my sister and I debated the pros and cons of telling everyone at that moment or waiting until the following week. We decided my office was going to find out anyway, so what did it matter if it was today? Did I mention we were *action* people yet? People will probably be shocked by what I did next. Out of the blue, I called five or six folks into my office and told them I had breast cancer. Yep—found out at 2:00 p.m., and my office knew by 2:30 p.m. I'm not kidding. I look back on that decision now, and even I'm shocked I thought it was a good idea. After stunning folks into silence, I proceeded home. I called my primary care clinician for a list of surgical oncologists, and I cried and cried and cried.

Then came the next "announcement" decision: how do I tell everyone else? I decided an e-mail and a Facebook post was appropriate. Yep— that was my thought process: I should post "I have cancer" on Facebook. But before posting on Facebook, I set up a blog.

I highly recommend keeping a blog. You will find yourself answering the same questions unless you just send out information for everyone to see. The blog site I used also allowed me to schedule "help" from my friends and family. This "help" was essential to my fight. My sister and her family are my nearest relatives, and they live about a three-hour drive away. My parents are retired and live in Florida, and my fiancé was not living locally at the time. My friends were my local support. They prepared meals, drove me to appointments, and kept my spirits lifted.

My blog kept everyone, including my long distance friends and relatives, in the loop and up-to-date. I can't underestimate the importance.

My blog posts were the foundation for this book, and my friends and family were my encouragement to write it. I used the site called MyLifeLine.org, and a friend of mine used CaringBridge.org. There are probably other sites as well. Explore them for yourself, or maybe this is the first opportunity to enlist the help of your family and friends.

Oh, by the way, if you're curious, here's my actual Facebook post.

I've set up a blog.

http://www.mylifeline.org

Most of you will be asking why … I wish it were better news, but on Friday I was diagnosed with breast cancer, specifically invasive ductal carcinoma. I know everyone will have lots of questions. My blog will hopefully keep everyone informed of my progress and answer questions. It all happened very, very fast.

My treatment will be surgery, chemo, and radiation—the extent of each is unknown until I receive information from a few more tests.

The support I've received this week is amazing! I intend to kick cancer's a$$! Please visit my blog. :-)

Yep—my "I have cancer" Facebook post was a winner. This may not be the best approach for everyone, but for me it was a great way to get the word out quickly, stop fussing about how to tell folks, and start kicking cancer's ass!

Most of my family and friends understand my craziness and were not completely shocked by a Facebook post. I am blessed!

This is a good time to also talk about the support I received in my office. I wish for everyone the same assistance and support. For example, right before I went out for surgery, my office threw me a *surprise* "Go Kick Cancer's Ass Party"! I *love* my office. One of the women even braved the bus and metro with a fantastic cake. I'm sure it was a spectacle as she juggled her coffee and a very large cake. Apparently, she visited at least two bakeries where she asked to have "Kick Cancer's Ass" written on the cake. "Ass" is not allowed on a cake! Who knew there were cake police? This party was exactly what I needed before heading to surgery and recovery.

In addition to celebrating the small victories and keeping my spirits lifted, my leadership offered even more support by allowing me to work from home during chemotherapy. This eliminated my commute and limited my contact with germs. I can't say enough good things about my staff, my coworkers, and my leadership. The stars aligned for me. I truly hope they align for everyone fighting this battle.

Unsolicited Advice

Most folks want to help, so let them help! Set up a blog or other information highway to keep family and friends informed. In addition, don't be afraid to ask for special considerations in your workplace. You're going to need a lot of flexibility!

Chapter 2

Action–Get Organized

(Standing in the office supply store, we were staring at a wall of binders ...)

Me: "Wow—that's a lot of choices."

Sister: "Well, what are you planning to store in the binder?"

Me: "Hmm ... probably questions for the doctor, telephone numbers, and medical records."

Sister: "Okay. You need to be able to add to it, so we can eliminate spiral bound binders."

Me: (silence) "Maybe I can choose the color first. I like this purple one."

Sister: "Seriously? That binder will hold about three sheets of paper!"

Me: "I need a new pen" (said as I walked away ...).

(An hour later, we walked out with the "perfect" binder and pen!)

THOSE WHO KNOW ME understand I have a plan for everything. (And for the record, cancer was not in my plan ...) So, once I worked through my initial meltdown, my instincts took over, and I started planning. Luckily for me, the planning craziness runs in the family.

My sister hopped in the car and headed my way within a couple of hours of hearing my cancer news. I was so grateful for her visit. First, she was with me as I worked through a bunch of initial emotions, and since she's my sister, she knows all my craziness. Second, she's an extreme planner!

The day after my diagnosis, we were cruising stores in search of the perfect filing, note taking, and information system. Oh, and I mean *system*. For extreme planners, such as the Bontempos, this means analyzing every option and debating the pros and cons of the 1-inch verses the 1.5-inch binder.

I bet all you non-planners are scared! I am happy to report that we settled on two notebooks. The first was a 1.5-inch binder, complete with business card pages, pocket pages, and dividers. This notebook was used to catalogue benefits statements from the insurance company and to keep all my info in one place. I can't begin to count the number of benefits statements, bills, and refund checks that I received during this fight. I highly recommend organizing from the beginning. Insurance companies and billing departments make mistakes. You need your information in one place in order to recognize the mistakes and have them corrected. Don't be afraid to call. I found the billing departments very willing to answer questions and work with me on payment options.

In addition, I picked up business cards from all the doctors. I always had the numbers handy and yes, I did include one or two in my speed dial.

The second notebook was smaller, and I carried it every day to jot down to-do lists and to take notes during phone calls. There were *a lot* of phone calls.

After getting my notebooks in order, it was time to set up my "Cancer Command Center." A lot of folks who visited my condo commented about it, which always made me laugh. We even decided "C3" was an appropriate acronym. Let me try to describe the area.

The necessary components of my Cancer Command Center were as follows:

- Comfy couch—the comfy couch also housed a kitty bed for those moments when I could convince my constant cat companion to be more than six inches from me (it was not often).
- Prayer shawl—I received two prayer shawls, which were both within easy reach for rapid deployment when needed.
- Cancer quilt—a friend made an awesome cancer quilt, which was my constant security blanket through this fight.
- Coffee table—the coffee table was of an adequate size to hold the remaining items:
  - computer
  - iPad
  - Kindle
  - chargers for the computer, iPad, and Kindle
  - 1.5-inch cancer binder and a three-hole punch for additions to the 1.5-inch binder
  - cancer books (lots and lots of cancer books)
  - pictures of the family and friends

Also within a short reach were wine and liquor, but that's another story.

Unsolicited Advice

Get organized for whatever is thrown your way! Call the billing departments with any questions, and don't be afraid to ask for flexibility!

Chapter 3

Action—Meet the Doctors,
Learn the Vocabulary, and Get
Ready for New Experiences

Me: "You are not going to believe this."

Sister: "What?"

Me: "I was face down for the breast MRI."

Sister: "What?"

Me: "Yep. I had to lie face down while the MRI tech stuffed
my boobs into two holes and then crawled underneath the
machine to position them!"

Sister: "What?"

Me: "I'm not kidding! And the holes weren't that large, so there
was a lot of 'positioning'!"

B REAST CANCER PROVIDED SO many new words for my vocabulary
and new experiences to enrich my life. First, I had to get used to
saying *breasts*, *boobs*, and *tatas*. I said the words more in the first month of
diagnosis than I had in my entire forty-one years! And … the number
of people who touched, prodded, and examined said breasts, boobs, and
tatas in the first month far exceeded recent memory! This is why my
sister recommended investing in Mardi Gras beads. Yes, Mardi Gras
beads. It became a dare (and a joke) for me to carry the beads in my
purse to the appointments. Once I was done showing my boobs to the
next set of strangers, I was dared to whip out my beads and wear them

through the doctor's waiting room. I'm sorry to say, I didn't actually follow through on the dare, but maybe you will be sassy enough to do it!

One of my first new phrases was *surgical oncologist*. This was the doctor who removed the damn cancer! This was, in other words, the doctor who performed my lumpectomy.

My doctors were wonderful! My initial meeting with the surgical oncologist lasted close to ninety minutes and included explaining and answering ... then explaining more ... and answering more. In order to make an informed decision about a lumpectomy, mastectomy, or double mastectomy, more information was still needed after the initial visit. For me, this involved the "receptor" information results from the biopsy to determine what made the cancer grow (estrogen, for example), an MRI to receive even more information about the size and location of the tumor, and an exciting visit with a plastic surgeon.

I scheduled my MRI within a day or two of my visit with the surgical oncologist. I was not looking forward to stuffing myself into a tube for forty-five minutes ... *breathe! Breathe! Breathe!*

But as you know from the exchange with my sister, I was face down with my breasts stuffed into two holes for the MRI. My head rested "comfortably" in a massage table headrest, but ... did you read the last sentence? My breasts were stuffed into two holes ... and ... they were placed there "gently" by the MRI tech! Who knew? The results showed more detail on the tumor and confirmed nothing was missed in the mammogram or the ultrasound.

The receptor information was available the week following my visit with the surgical oncologist. I had an estrogen and progesterone receptive cancer. Apparently, if you're going to get breast cancer, this is the one to get. There are more treatment options for this type of receptor, and lucky me, I will be taking a pill for the next five to ten years to keep estrogen levels moderated. Intellectually, I understand this is a good thing, and the fact I have the option is amazing, but I can hardly remember to take a multivitamin once per day.

I also met with a plastic surgeon and joked with my friends about having a plastic surgeon on speed dial. I never expected to be visiting a plastic surgeon, but I looked at the bright side and dreamed of nipping this and tucking that. Yep—this attitude is all part of my silver lining personality.

Again, I *never* thought I'd end up at a plastic surgeon. Yes, I have body issues, everyone does, but they were never such a big deal as to drive me to a plastic surgeon's office (although I admit, I thought about it …). Well, point one for cancer: I now have a plastic surgeon. For my lumpectomy, the plastic surgeon operated with the surgical oncologist and "reshaped" my breast after the tumor was removed. My left breast was now perkier and "smaller" from removing the cancer.

I met a couple of friends for lunch following the MRI and plastic surgeon appointments to relay my stories. They expressed exactly the right amount of shock, horror, and bewilderment at the absurdity of my situation. Then we headed for wine.

Take some time to enjoy yourself as you go though this. It's important to remember who you are and that cancer does not define you. I reminded myself of this often through lunches, dinners, and wine with family and friends.

This was also about the time I started seriously stressing about losing my hair. I was convinced I had aged about five years in the ten days following diagnosis and began noticing a *lot* of gray hair. Normally, I would have scheduled an appointment with my stylist, and she would have just taken care of it (she's a slayer of gray hair). But, with the "chemo cloud" hanging over my head, I was leery to color my hair and then promptly have it all fall out! In the end, I decided I wanted a little normalcy and that it would make me feel better to have it colored. So off I went for a cut and color—and yes, about two months later, it all fell out! However, I do not regret this indulgence. I was still me—and

I needed to keep my life normal. As simple as it seems, having my hair cut and colored allowed me a day of normalcy. Take the time to keep your life normal.

Now is a good time to take one moment to tell you about genetic testing. I've decided to use my blog on the subject to spread the word. Enjoy!

Do My Genes Fit? The Story of Genetic Testing!

I do not have the "cancer gene"!

If you are asking yourself, "What's the cancer gene?" you are not alone! Up until my diagnosis, the words *cancer* and *gene* would not have been used in the same sentence, but here I am about to give you the 101.

While at the appointment with the surgical oncologist, she mentioned that the genetic counselor was in the office and asked if I'd like to speak with her. *Huh? Sure ... okay ...* (I really didn't know what she meant, but I thought, why not?)

As it turns out, a lot of research has pinpointed two genes that, when mutations are present, significantly increase the risk of a woman developing breast cancer. The genes are called BRCA1 and BRCA2. The genetic test is performed for a couple of reasons. First, if a woman has a history of breast cancer in her family, this test can confirm if the gene is present and therefore be used for prevention options, such as six-month mammograms.

In my case, there was no family history. However, if the mutation is present in a woman who has breast cancer, there is a sixty percent chance that the cancer will reappear in the other breast! With odds like that, I wanted to know!

The actual test was interesting. No swabs or blood! I was handed a small bottle of mouthwash. I was then asked to swish the mouthwash in my mouth and spit into a tube. I then ran my tongue around my teeth and again spit into the tube. I then sealed the tube, and off it went for genetic testing. I left the office with minty fresh breath!

Approximately ten days later, the genetic counselor called with the good news. This was the last bit of information I needed to be completely sure of my decision for a lumpectomy.

Unsolicited Advice

Read books, research online, and start learning the vocabulary. It makes communicating with doctors and nurses much easier! Don't forget to take the time to relax and keep your life normal!

Chapter 4

Action—Take Control

Me: "I'm going crazy!"

Sister: "You're just realizing this?"

Me: "Very funny. I'm serious. My life is out of control! Help! What are you up to?"

Sister: "Well, let's see. I have two four-year-olds screaming in timeout. They decided they wanted a lake in the living room. I'm trying to borrow fans from my neighbors to dry out the upstairs and downstairs carpets. At the moment, I'm tearing down the basement ceiling where the water leaked through. So tell me again how your life is out of control?"

Me: (silence). "Maybe I'll call back later. Thanks for the laugh! Good luck with the cleanup."

I LOVED MY SURGICAL ONCOLOGIST and the nurses and staff! But the hospital system was a little frustrating at times. A couple of weeks after my initial visit with the surgical oncologist, I still did not have a surgery date.

My meltdowns, my sarcastic e-mails, and my telephone messages were not working. I was trying very hard to be patient, but cancer was growing inside me, and I wanted it out! It was time for me to become my own advocate.

After complaining and complaining and enduring a complete lack of sleep, I wrote a nasty e-mail dripping with sarcasm and self-pity. Luckily for me, I still had an ounce of sanity left, and I sent it off to my sister for editing. She magically converted nastiness and sarcasm into a firm, inquisitive, and appropriate e-mail. Okay—so she let me keep a little of my self-pity and sarcasm … I know you're curious, so here's an excerpt.

> I'm 100 percent completely and utterly stressed about not having surgery scheduled. When you speak to the scheduler, please reminder her I'm the one with cancer. I'm the one who's not sleeping. I'm the one who looks in the mirror every morning and realizes that I am no closer to beating cancer today than I was yesterday. Frustrating is an understatement. I want this cancer out of my body. There is a real person on the other side of this e-mail who is terrified, angry, and feels helpless. I am not a tumor, and I am not a block of time.

There was more, but this gives you the idea. I sent it off, and surgery was scheduled! I was thrilled to have the surgery date, and this was a huge lesson. Be your own advocate. There will be times when you will need to be firm to ensure you receive the care you need. Just do it. You won't be sorry.

Here's your public service announcement for this chapter. If you receive news that you have an estrogen and progesterone receptive cancer, it is not advisable to stick with hormonal birth control; basically, stop taking the pill or anything that resembles the pill. Lucky me, I added the gynecologist to the list of folks poking and prodding me during this time. Non-hormonal birth control options are limited to the IUD and stuff you can buy in the grocery store. Who knew? There is an option if the cancer is *just* estrogen receptive, but mine was not. My cancer was both estrogen and progesterone receptive. Since getting pregnant was not an option while going through cancer treatments, I also added this to the list of craziness that was thrown at me all at once.

Unsolicited Advice

Take control, and be your own advocate! This is your journey and your fight. Call, beg, plead, visit, and stomp your feet until you have the answers you need and the schedule you want!

Chapter 5

Action–Embrace the Emotional Hurricane

Me: "I bought a new car today."

Sister: "What? A real car or one for the boys?"

Me: "I left the office early and bought one for me."

Sister: "Of course you did ..."

Me: "And I cried with the car salesman."

Sister: "What? Please tell me he gave you a good deal."

Me: "Yes, he did, but I'm a basket case, and I cried with my new best friend the car salesman."

Sister: "Okay ... congratulations?" (Even over the phone, I could hear the question and confusion in her voice.)

IT'S HARD TO EXPLAIN the emotions that came tumbling into my brain when I was told I had breast cancer. I was shocked; I was angry; I was terrified; and that was just the beginning of this emotional hurricane.

Here is one of my blogs to give you an idea of my emotions within three weeks of my diagnosis.

Introspective Rambling

Being stuck in my house for three days forced me to embrace my cancer! Well, maybe *embrace* is the wrong word, but I had very few distractions and therefore thought about it *a lot* ... I've come to a few conclusions.

1. Cancer sucks!

As an information gatherer, I have spent way too much time over the last few days pouring through books on cancer. Some of them are real downers! I must admit, they are full of information, but wow, they are not a fun read. Where are the sarcastic, educational cancer books?

2. Cancer college is no fun!

As I read through all of these books, I felt as if I were back in school. I liked school; I loved college; I even enjoyed my master's program. So why is cancer college so different? It's not just academic; it's my life! Holy crap! Everything I read impacts me directly and immediately! That's a lot pressure to put on a girl!

3. I have no patience!

Okay—I knew this before cancer. Waiting for surgery is a real drag. I want action! I'll probably long for these days once I wake up from surgery, but right now, it's just painful!

4. I like my job, and it pisses me off that I have to slow down!

We're in the middle of deploying software. I've told my coworkers that I feel as if I signed up for a marathon, and at mile twenty-five I'm being told I have to drop out of the race. Are you kidding me? It pisses me off. If I have to fight cancer, I want to do it on my terms and on my schedule. Guess what? I don't have that luxury! It's so unfair!

5. Life is unfair!

This was just one blog entry, but emotional hurricane stories were plentiful during this journey. For example, I decided to buy a car three days before my lumpectomy. Why? I have no idea! But, I believe some people come into your life for a reason: to teach you something, to make you appreciate something, or to just make you smile when you don't feel like smiling. I *never* expected an Acura salesman to be one of those folks!

I had been in the market for a new car for a few months. The Acura was my car of choice, and I decided three days before my lumpectomy was the perfect time to buy it ... so I headed over to the Acura dealership and met Ed for the first time. Ed found me in the parking lot as I was walking through the sea of Acuras. Over the next hour we test drove two cars and sat in probably ten. I decided on this *awesome* black exterior, black interior model, and we headed inside for the paperwork.

He was making small talk and asked if my family lived close, as Thanksgiving was a week away. I looked him in the eye, and after only a *brief* pause, I told him that I was diagnosed with breast cancer and that my surgery was Monday, so I would be missing out on Thanksgiving with my family (of course I did—who does this?). He told me that every year he raises money for breast cancer research and participates in the Race for the Cure.

We then proceeded with the rest of the deal. Yes, I got a great deal, but that was not the story.

As he opened the door of my car, he grabbed both my hands and looked me in the eye. He said, "I have known many women who have fought breast cancer and won. You are going to win."

I told him he was going to make me cry, and then tears started running down my face. His eyes also filled with tears. Again he reiterated that I would beat cancer, and then he asked for a hug.

Who does this? I had a crying, hugging moment with my car salesman! Can you say emotional hurricane?

Unsolicited Advice

You are in for an emotional hurricane. Embrace it! Cry, yell, cry some more, scream, do whatever you want! This is your fight, and your emotions are exactly what they should be!

Part 2

Breast Surgery

Me: "I wonder how many more people will see my breasts during surgery."
Sister: "Just remember: it's like Mardi Gras. You keep showing your boobs to strangers."
Me: "Sure—it's just like Mardi Gras, but without the alcohol or the fun!"

THE "SHORTEST" PART OF my journey involved my lumpectomy. My surgery was five weeks after diagnosis, with two weeks of recovery. I still had some pain after two weeks, but I was able to wear a bra, which I translated to "I was able to get back to my life and even go to work."

Finding out I needed surgery was scary. I despise being stuck with needles and get woozy at the sight of blood. The whole medical experience is pretty miserable for everyone because I'm usually nervous and scared when someone tries to "stick me." Therefore, it takes numerous "sticks." I only tell you this to prepare you for the next few chapters. If you are one of those lucky folks who can easily give blood and have an IV inserted, you will probably not have significant problems with this phase of your treatment.

Chapter 6

Action—Brace Yourself
for the Unknown

Me: "The plastic surgeon took pictures of my boobs today."
Sister: (silence) "Did you ask for a pink boa so you could send
    the pictures to your fiancé?"
Me: "Damn—I should have!"

THE WEEK PRIOR TO surgery, I met with both the surgical oncologist
and the plastic surgeon.

The appointment with the plastic surgeon was way more interesting.
The 1980s song "Centerfold" by the J. Geils Band jumped into my
head when the assistant at the plastic surgeon's office told me to "strip
from the waist up, and we'll take some pictures." I'm not kidding! This
would have been a fantastic appointment to whip out my Mardi Gras
beads and proudly wear them for photos.

My plastic surgeon was in surgery when I arrived for my pre-operation
visit. As I was escorted into an exam room to await his arrival, his
assistant started the conversation with, "Strip from the waist up, and
we'll take some pictures." (You'd better be singing "Centerfold" by
now!) I'm sure she noticed the shocked look on my face. *Are you kidding?*
Again, I should have seen this coming, but I didn't. I laughed when I
thought of my fiancé, who had been asking for these pictures for years,

and here I was about to undress for a complete stranger to take pictures of my boobs!

When she returned, I was dutifully stripped from the waist up and covered in a robe. As she entered, I noticed the backdrop on the wall behind me. Thank goodness it wasn't some fall scene with a stream running through it or, even worse, a velvet couch! It looked more like a passport photo location. She then proceeded to ask me to "stand straight," "turn to the right," "turn to the left," and my favorite, "place your hands behind your back and stand up straight"! Oh—the absurdity. I started laughing and asked the young woman, "Do you really take pictures of boobs all day?" "Yep," she said and started laughing. At least she didn't hand me a boa!

I did inquire if I would *ever* have to look at these photos. She said probably not as she walked out the door, adding, "I'm going to print these and put them in your file now." Oh, geez!

And this was only the beginning of my boob modeling adventures. There are boob photos in my file with the plastic surgeon, the medical oncologist, the radiation oncologist, and probably a few more I can't remember at the moment. Boob photos—brace yourself; there were a lot of boob photos!

Unsolicited Advice

Expect the unexpected. There will be many days when you "discover" situations, such as boob photos. Go with the flow, and keep your sense of humor!

Chapter 7

Action–Relax and Breathe; Surgery Day Has Arrived

Sister: "Good luck with surgery tomorrow!"

Me: "I've been reading about this needle localization thing."

Sister: "Why?"

Me: "At first, because I wanted to be prepared ... and now because I'm mortified. Supposedly wires will be sticking out of my breast! WTF! I picture some alien abduction gone wrong!"

Sister: (silence) "Are you allowed to drink alcohol tonight?"

Me: "I mean, seriously. Picture this ... I'm in a hospital bed with wires sticking out of my breast and an IV in my arm. If I see a wire or two sticking out of my breast, I'm running for the hills, fainting, or laughing hysterically ... your guess is as good as mine as to which one! I could end up in a loony bin!"

Sister: "I'll come and bust you out if you end up in a loony bin, and I'll bring alcohol."

I RECEIVED A SURGERY CHECKLIST from the surgical oncologist's office about a week before surgery. There was an entry for "needle localization" prior to the lumpectomy. Hmmmm ... okay ... what's a needle localization? Off to the Internet I went! (What did we do before the Internet???)

Scary! Scary! Scary! Here's what the Komen website (www.komen.org) had to say! "A procedure called wire-localization or needle-localization will be done before surgery. A radiologist uses a mammogram, ultrasound or MRI as a guide and inserts a very thin wire into the breast in the area of the cancer. The surgeon then uses this wire as a guide to find and remove the tumor during surgery."

Say what? And guess what? I would be awake while they stuck a wire into my breast! No general anesthesia until after this fun and exciting procedure.

So let's talk about the day of surgery. I arrived at the hospital at 8:00 a.m., as instructed. We were very efficiently moved through registration and into the pre-op waiting area. The friendly nurse inserted an IV. As we were heading off to the needle localization around 9:00 a.m., the nurse walked out to check the schedule. Nope, it wouldn't be at 9:00 a.m. ... not at 10:00 a.m. either. The needle localization was scheduled for 11:00 a.m. Great. Here it was, 9:00 a.m.; I had an IV stuck in the back of my hand and another two hours to wait.

So we waited ... and around 11:00 a.m., I was wheeled down to radiology for the needle localization. This procedure was archaic! Someone should come up with something better! And it freakin' *hurt!* Basically, they pressed me into a mammogram machine with a hole in one of the plates. Once I was "immobilized," they stuck a needle through the hole and then a wire through the needle. All the while, they took images to be sure the needle and the wire were sticking in the tumor. It was insane! There was lots of crying during this fun, little procedure. But the wires were taped to my skin, so I didn't faint or run for the hills. I did, however, get mad because it sucked so bad, *and* there were no Mardi Gras beads! After it was completed, they wheeled me back to pre-op to wait another two hours for surgery.

So we waited ... and about ten minutes before the surgery, a nurse arrived to put something in my IV. It hurt so bad, I about jumped off the bed! My IV was compromised. By this time, I was scared, I was cold, and I was in pain. The nurse spent the next ten minutes trying to insert another IV. I had five more holes and five more black and blue marks, but no IV. The anesthesiologist came in and suggested we knock me out through the mask in the operating room and then insert the IV. I was all for that plan.

So they wheeled me into the operating room. It was strange being awake in an operating room, but my thoughts immediately jumped to the beads I should be collecting given all the folks in the room. A few deep breaths through the mask, and I was out.

The next thing I remember, I was waking up in recovery. Apparently, the first time they woke me up, I was in enough pain that the nurses gave me a sedative and put me back to sleep for two hours. It was somewhere in the neighborhood of 7:00 p.m. when I woke up and was able to go home.

As part of my lumpectomy, the surgical oncologist removed a total of five lymph nodes. They tested the lymph nodes for cancer, and the results were available immediately. Two tested positive for the cancer, so chemotherapy was definitely in my future.

However, I chose to also celebrate. Of the five lymph nodes removed, three did not have cancer! Again, this is just part of my silver lining personality. I also needed a little celebration after my IV needle experience.

Unsolicited Advice

I repeat. Expect the unexpected. Go with the flow, and keep your sense of humor!

Chapter 8

Action—Get to Those Follow-Up Appointments!

Me: "I hate this drain!"

Sister: "I can't even imagine."

Me: "This is the best option we have in 2012? A plastic hose connected to a plastic bottle that sucks crap out of my chest ...? It's disgusting!"

Sister: (laughing). "Yep."

IN MY LUMPECTOMY, IT was necessary to install a drain to allow the fluid to drain from my chest. During the follow-up with my plastic surgeon, the annoying, irritating, wretched, pesky drain was removed! If you couldn't tell from the last sentence, I was so excited to be rid of the hose that stuck out of my chest and emptied into a plastic bottle pinned to my bra. Who came up with this thing?

I was also cleared to switch from Percocet to Motrin, which meant I was able to drive. In addition, the plastic surgeon knew me well enough to say I could have a glass of wine in a couple of days. I was thrilled at the end of this appointment.

This was also the beginning of my ongoing battle with allergic reactions to drugs and the resulting rashes. In this case, the rash was on my arms, chest, and stomach. The surgeon and I concluded this was probably an allergic reaction to either the antibiotic or the Percocet. I stopped taking both and started on Benadryl for a few days. The rash cleared up in less than a week.

I also met with the surgical oncologist to hear all the details about my tumor. First, the pathology results showed I had *"clean margins."* Although this may sound as though I didn't spill coffee on a term paper, in the cancer world this was good news for much more significant reasons. Basically, when they removed the tumor, they checked the pathology along the outside of the tumor. They measured the space between the cancer and the edge of the removed area—this space is called "the margin." If there is no cancer in "the margins," this is referred to as "clean margins."

As I stated in the last chapter, the surgical oncologist removed five lymph nodes during the lumpectomy. Unfortunately, two tested positive for cancer. I hate cancer!

My tumor also ended up being *much* larger than expected. The MRI imagery showed the tumor at 1.9 centimeters by 1.7 centimeters by 1.4 centimeters. The tumor was *actually* 4 centimeters by 3.5 centimeters by 1.3 centimeters! And ... they *removed* 6 centimeters by 6 centimeters by 3.5 centimeters! Now that was a *big* difference. Apparently the imagery was not as crystal clear as one might hope. No kidding!

The last follow-up appointment was with the physical therapist. I had great range of motion after the surgery and didn't need extended physical therapy. I only saw the physical therapist twice: once for the assessment and once for the lymphedemia session and sleeve fitting. Lymphedemia is possible if you have lymph nodes removed and can affect the arm closest to the lymph node removal site. Several folks will talk to you about the specifics, but wearing the sleeve and being cautious about cuts on the affected arm is the best way to minimize your risk. This also means you should always use the unaffected arm when having your blood pressure checked, having blood drawn, or receiving an IV. It's easy once you get used to it.

There is one more blog entry for this section. Although I chose a lumpectomy, I researched and asked questions about mastectomies and double mastectomies. During my research, I discovered Vinnie. Here's my blog entry with more info.

Vinnie from Baltimore

Some of my blogs are intended to be educational. This cancer thing is *all* new to me, and wow, am I learning more than I ever wanted to know about the subject! This is one of those blogs. :-)

I am clueless in certain areas ... hmm ... many areas ... but I digress. In this blog, I'm specifically addressing my cluelessness with regard to mastectomies and nipples. (Yep—you read that correctly.) I did not realize that in the vast majority of cases, nipples are removed during the mastectomy. Okay—it makes sense, but I never thought about it!

There is a growing research area call "nipple sparing" surgery, but at the moment, it is limited to women with "smaller" breasts.

Okay, back to the point. Once I had this piece of information, I thought *crap!* ... and then I needed to know more! I'm not going to lie; I was freaked out by it (as if you couldn't tell that from this blog). And so ... nipples were one of the topics of conversation with my surgical oncologist.

My doctor told me about "Vinnie from Baltimore," who travels around the country tattooing. I burst out laughing, and then I started crying! Vinnie from Baltimore sounded like a bad movie! And my conversation about nipples seemed so absurd! Seriously? Are you kidding me? Someone makes a living tattooing nipples? Yep—and apparently he is one of the best in the country. I won't include his webpage here because some of you may be viewing this blog with your United States

Government computers. But, I have visited his site, and I've made several of my friends look at it too. :-)

Unsolicited Advice

Get to those follow-up appointments! First, it might lift your spirits when you are able to stop the meds and have the drains removed. Second, you need all the information from the follow-up appointments to make the next set of decisions. This is also when you probably will need the help of family and friends, as you won't be able to drive.

Part 3

Chemotherapy

Sister: "How are you feeling today?"
Me: "Like I was hit by a bus."
Sister: "Hang in there. You'll get through this. There is light at
the end of the tunnel"
Me: (silence) "Yep, but I'm afraid that light is the train about
to hit me!"

I'M JUST GOING TO state it up front: chemotherapy sucked! My lumpectomy was November 19, and less than one month later, I started chemo. Four long months later, I finished. Everyone's experience is unique and my doctors explained my chemo was unusually bad, but expect to hate chemotherapy. I've tried in the next few chapters to give you some unsolicited advice for dealing with chemo and the emotions inevitably that hit you like a hurricane during this phase. Hang in there! Once this phase was complete, I felt like a superhero—capable of beating anything!

Chapter 9

Action—Meet More Doctors and Learn More Vocabulary

Me: "I met with the medical oncologist today."

Sister: "What did she say?"

Me: "The next four months are going to suck."

Sister: "Yep. Anything else?"

Me: "The next four months are going to suck. Did she need to say anything else?"

Sister: (silence)

Me: "I have to go to chemo class."

Sister: "Is there a test at the end?"

Me: "Huh?"

Sister: "Are they going to test you on your chemo knowledge?"

Me: "I don't think so."

Sister: "Good, because you won't get an A with the answer 'The next four months are going to suck!'"

BECAUSE CANCER CELLS WERE found in two of my lymph nodes, another doctor was added to the growing list in my care circle—a medical oncologist. This was the doctor in charge of the chemotherapy portion of my treatment. My initial meeting with the medical oncologist lasted close to sixty minutes and included explaining the benefits of chemotherapy and walking through the expected side effects. In my head I bolted for the hills several times, but physically, I stayed put and listened intently.

In my case, the doctor recommended six rounds of the drug combination known as TAC (Taxotere, Adriamycin, and Cytoxan). The six rounds were to be delivered once every three weeks. As it turns out, I experienced a reaction to the Taxotere and switched to the drug Taxol after only one treatment, but more on that later.

Let's get back to the side effects as I knew them *before* I started chemo. The doctor explained I could expect two major side effects:

- losing my hair
- fatigue

She also listed eight or ten additional possible side effects and stated that I'd most likely have one or two of those. I looked at the list. Wow—some were better than others ... but as with everything else with cancer, this was out of my control, and I didn't get to choose my side effects. That lack of control was tough throughout this fight. If you have looked ahead to the next few chapters, you already know that I had more than one or two of the ones she listed.

As I mentioned previously, I experienced a reaction to the Taxotere during my first infusion, and within a week, my doctor switched chemo drugs. Unfortunately for me, the new chemo cocktail was administered every two weeks (instead of every three weeks), and I needed eight infusions (instead of six). Boo! Hiss! I had just wrapped my head around chemo every three weeks, when everything changed. While intellectually I understood this was the best course of action, I was *not* (*not! not! not! not! not!*) looking forward to going through chemo every two weeks. In the end, my regimen was one round of TAC, followed by three rounds of AC (Adriamycin and Cytoxan), followed by four rounds of Taxol.

For even more information after my initial visit with the medical oncologist, the office offered a chemo class. The class was very informative! It lasted two hours and included information about side effects, resources, and telephone numbers. I took my mom with me to chemo class, and I recommend taking someone with you. I was freaked out, and it helped having someone less freaked out taking notes.

Unsolicited Advice

Meet the doctors, and pay close attention! If the office offers a chemo class, take it! My doctors (and nurses) answered a ton of questions leading up to chemo. Don't be afraid to ask!

Chapter 10

Action–Get to Those
Appointments!

Me: "I'm overwhelmed."
Sister: "About what?"
Me: "All of these appointments before chemo."
Sister: "Do you want help?"
Me: "Well, no. I just want to complain."
Sister: (silence)
Me: "Okay, maybe I could use some help."
Sister: "Excellent! What do you need?"
Me: (silence) "You know I'm not actually going to take the
   help, right?"
Sister: "Ugh ..."
Me: "I'll tell folks to accept the help when I write my book."
Sister: "You should take your own advice."
Me: "Probably ..."

THERE WAS A WHIRLWIND of activity between my lumpectomy and
the start of chemo. My Mardi Gras bead tally continued to grow
as I endured yet more procedures. For me, this included

- a CT scan,
- an echocardiogram, and

- a fun and exciting procedure to install a port—more on this in a minute.

The CT Scan

Yep—I had never had a CT scan. I drank a lot of barium for this procedure. I woke up at 5:30 a.m. to drink one bottle; I drank half of a second bottle at 6:30 a.m. and the remainder at 7:00 a.m. Then, I had another cup once I was at the CT scan at 7:30 a.m. That's a lot of barium! There is one interesting thing about this procedure. They hooked me up to an IV and administered iodine (I think it's for contrast). The iodine gave me a metallic taste in my mouth, and my entire body felt warm. It was very weird! All in all, this procedure was relatively easy.

The Echocardiogram

Yep—I had gone forty-one years without an echocardiogram either. In case you don't know (I didn't), an echocardiogram is an ultrasound of your heart. Several chemotherapy drugs have been linked to heart issues, so the medical oncologist wanted to be sure I didn't have an existing heart issue, and she wanted to establish a baseline before chemotherapy. It was a very simple procedure where I lounged on my back and on my side while they rolled the ultrasound wand over my heart. This was just one more procedure where I was showing my boobs to strangers, and yes, I was thinking of Mardi Gras beads. The only weird thing about this procedure was that I was able to hear my heartbeat. It's kind of freaky to hear your own heart beating.

The Fun and Exciting Procedure to Install the Port

The port is another one of those entertaining devices I knew nothing about before this cancer thing. To eliminate the need for an IV each time chemotherapy is administered, a small device (about the size of a quarter and the thickness of my finger) was installed near my collarbone. The port was installed beneath the skin, and a tube (catheter) connected the port to a vein in my neck. This allowed the chemo drugs to be injected directly into the vein with less discomfort than the typical "needle stick" and IV.

So let me see if I can explain the procedure to install the port. This was an outpatient procedure lasting a couple of hours. Since I was knocked out partially with narcotics, I needed someone to drive me to and from the procedure. (Get your peeps lined up! You'll need help with transportation for this one.) First I needed an IV. I tried to warn folks that my veins did not like to cooperate with IVs and that I was usually scared, which made the situation worse. However, everyone wanted to give it a try. Nurse number one tried once and said, "I'll go get someone else." Nurse number two tried twice. Nurse number three—woo hoo! Let's hear it for nurse number three, who installed the IV successfully. Next, they wheeled me into the operating room for the procedure. Since I was only in "twilight" sedation, not full general anesthesia, they tented my head while they installed the port. It was very strange. I couldn't see what they were doing, but I was in and out of sleep during the procedure and dreamed of crazy Mardi Gras beads. Once the procedure was complete, I was as good as new within a couple of hours. The port itself was removed about six months later. For me, removing the port was another reason for a celebration to mark the end of chemo! One of my friends named her port while she went through chemo. I referred to mine as the "damn port," but be creative! You'll alternately love and hate this thing for six months.

Unsolicited Advice

Get to all those pre-chemo appointments. If so inclined, name your new port friend!

Chapter 11

*Action–Take Control
(All about the Hair, Part One)*

Me: "I'm going to lose my hair."

Sister: "Yep."

Me: "I don't want to lose my hair."

Sister: "Nope."

Me: "What am I going to do?"

Sister: (silence) "Want me to come visit while you cut your hair short?"

Me: "I'm not exactly thinking about celebrating at the moment ..."

Sister: "We don't have to celebrate. We drink wine and cry if you want."

Me: (silence) "Hmm ... how about we throw a party?"

Sister: (silence) "Huh?"

Me: "A party would let me take back control, and I could donate my hair! Let's throw a party!"

Sister: "Okay. Let's throw a party."

Me: (singing into the phone) "It's my party, and I'll cry if I want to ..."

WITH EVERYTHING ELSE IN my life spiraling uncontrollably, I decided to take back a little control with a hair-cutting party. I invited about fifteen of my girlfriends for a Saturday afternoon celebration with champagne, wine, and, yes, some tears as I donated my hair to "Locks of Love." The only catch was that they had to tell me that my hair looked great. No matter what it looked like, my friends were instructed to tell me it looked fabulous!

As it turned out, this was a fantastic idea! I expected an emotional afternoon, but I was in for a shock. It was fun. Not only did I like the new hairdo, it was such a blast sharing the afternoon and evening with great friends.

So let me tell you about the time leading up to the party. The thing I dreaded most about chemo was losing my hair. I *loved* my hair. Initially, the thought of losing it scared the crap out of me. My hair was part of my identity. But the anticipation was way worse than actually losing it and being bald. My family and friends played a huge part in this. At every turn, they told me I looked great, and they told me I had a great head. Here's a piece of advice: tell someone you trust this little secret—whenever she sees you, she should tell you how awesome your bald head looks, and she should spread the word to your friends. I hope you see for yourself, it's not so bad to lose your hair. And hey, you save a ton of money on hair products and salon visits. Not to mention the time saved in the shower and prepping for leaving the house. Hang in there. You will get through this and probably build some confidence you didn't even know you needed.

As you can probably guess, I highly recommend doing something fun to mark this milestone. For me, it was a party. I also heard a great story of a woman who rented a convertible when her hair started to fall out. She drove seventy miles per hour down the highway with the wind whipping through her hair and the radio on full blast! I would have done this in a minute had I thought of it.

Unsolicited Advice

Do something fabulous before losing your hair!

Chapter 12

Action—Shake It Up (Wigs, Hats, Scarves, and Headbands!)

Me: "I'm single-handedly bringing back the headband for the
over-forty crowd."

Sister: (laughing) "What?"

Me: "I exercised my glue gun today and made a bunch of
headbands."

Sister: (still laughing) "Why?"

Me: "Think about it. I can use these headbands as hat accessories
and still be able to throw the hat in the washer. A whole new
world opened up to me today!"

Sister: "You know you are crazy right?"

Me: "Yep, but I'm accessorized ..."

LOSING MY HAIR OPENED up a whole new world of accessories. Yes,
that is a "silver lining" sentence. I didn't need a whole world of
accessories, but cancer had other ideas. So I decided to embrace the
craziness and adapt. I used wigs, hats, scarves, and headbands to show
my style (or lack thereof).

First, let me tell you about the wigs. Some insurance companies will
reimburse up to a certain amount if the doctor writes a prescription
for a "cranial prosthesis." I found this hysterical! But, I loved the

reimbursement from the insurance company. So back to wig shopping: oh, wig shopping ... this was another brand new experience. But, I put aside my apprehension and headed out wig shopping not long after I found out I would lose my hair. All the experts recommend shopping before you lose your hair, so you can match your style and color before your hair is gone.

I spent about ninety minutes trying on wigs the first visit. Holy crap, this was a weird experience. I highly recommend it, but expect to watch yourself change in the mirror with every wig. Some of the wigs looked good. Some of the wigs looked terrible! Until you try on about a zillion and a half, you won't know. In the end, I found one that remarkably matched the color and style of my hair prior to the haircutting celebration. Since my first visit was solo, I dragged my sister along before actually buying a wig. I found a second wig with her, which was a short, sassy style. I ended up buying them both.

Yes, I own two wigs, but I only ended up wearing them a couple of times. I felt much more comfortable in the hats, scarves, and headbands. This might be partly because of the timing of my chemo between December and March; hats were easy to wear in the cold weather. Whatever the case, do what makes *you* comfortable. However, don't miss out on the wig shopping experience and trying on a zillion and a half options.

Let's move on to the hats and scarves. There are so many hat and scarf options on the Internet and in local shops; you are going to find a few you love. A friend of mine was diagnosed about ten months before me, and she gifted me three bags of hats and scarves. I only needed to buy a few. There were a ton of options, and I found it kind of fun to shop for them. Go for it!

Lastly, my very own stylish option was making headbands for the hats. I discovered headbands could easily be used as hat accessories. I didn't want to add anything to the hats, which would limit throwing them in the washer and dryer, but adding a headband allowed me to accessorize.

I took this option to a whole new level with headbands of every color and style. Most of them I made myself with a glue gun and materials from craft stores.

Making the headbands is very easy. Start with store-bought cloth headbands in black and various colors—even the grocery stores carry these. Next let your imagination run wild. I used ribbon, paper flowers, and beads to create stylish options. I then wore the headbands over the hat, and poof: the same hat was transformed for unlimited options. The hat could still be thrown in the washer because nothing was attached directly to it! I received a ton of compliments (and comments) on the headbands. Go for it! Let your inner craft diva out.

Unsolicited Advice

Accessorize! Take this opportunity to let your imagination run wild with accessory options.

Chapter 13

Action–Take That Offer of Support (Chemo: The First Infusion)

Me: (talking very fast) "I think I'm ready for chemo tomorrow.
  I have a goody bag to take with me with snacks, my iPad, my
  Kindle, two magazines, and my iPhone."
Sister: (laughing) "What? I can barely understand you."
Me: (laughing) "I love these steroids! I'm not sleeping, but I'm
  getting a ton of stuff done."
Sister: (still laughing) "What?"
Me: "I only get to take the steroids for three days. I have to pack
  a month's worth of activity into three days."
Sister: (still laughing) "I think you are packing a month's worth
  of talking into three days!"
Me: "Probably. Gotta go!"

M Y MOM TRAVELED INTO town to accompany me to the first chemo
session and make sure I was well cared for during the days after.
She also had "the pleasure" of driving me to appointments, attending
chemo class with me, and "watching me like a hawk" for signs of
trouble. Moms and close friends are great for this kind of thing. I highly
recommend taking this offer of support.

I'll describe the first chemo session in a minute, but first, I want to talk about the best drug ever invented. I started taking a steroid the day before chemo. OMG—I *loved, loved, loved* this drug! I had so much energy, and my mental acuity felt like it was before I found out about the cancer. Unfortunately, I could only take the steroid for three days—something about long-term use and heart problems ... whatever, I *loved* it! Oh—and apparently the crash a couple of days after chemo was from both going off the steroid and from the chemo ... but whatever, I *loved* it! If you are lucky enough to be prescribed a steroid, take advantage of the energy.

Let's talk about the chemo infusion. Each session, I was seated in an infusion center with about five other folks. It was kind of like a very large, very sterile living room. There were groupings of two to four lounge chairs for patients to relax and sleep, as well as TVs, snacks, and drinks. Each lounge chair had its own IV pole and pump. The IV pole and pump could be moved if I needed to use the restroom (I asked immediately!), but for the most part, I sat in a lounge chair and chatted or browsed the Internet.

Once I picked a lounge chair, a friendly nurse came over to explain the process and the drugs. She also brought me ginger ale and a blanket, which made her my new BFF! She lost BFF status quickly, though, when I realized she was going to stick me in the port and hook me to an IV. It was a *large*, short needle for this stick. However, it wasn't very painful. As a matter of fact, it was much less painful than an IV, which made me thankful for the port. The nurse again was my BFF!

I received a bunch of pre-treatment drugs and the chemo drugs via IV during the infusion. Each required a different amount of time to go through the IV, so the nurses hooked me up and waited for the alarm. When the alarm sounded, the nurses came back and hooked me up to the next one. The last chemo drug was expected to take an hour, but they started me off with a short dosage, as sometimes folks have a reaction to it. If you recall from a previous chapter, I had a reaction. Yep, this is where it all happened. Abdominal cramps started shortly after the drug was administered. I, of course, rationalized the cramps were a result of something I ate. The nurses weren't buying the "something I ate" rationalization. So they added a little Benadryl, and we started again.

So this is where the story gets a little weird. I had altitude sickness in 2007, and this little reaction was very similar. In that instance, I was complaining of abdominal cramps prior to heading over a pass in the mountains of Montana. Then I turned green. In this case, I was pretty sure the tenth floor wasn't considered high enough for "altitude sickness," but wow—the reaction was very similar! The nurses again weren't buying my "altitude sickness" rationalization. It was just a plain old reaction to the chemo drug.

Mom and I ended up leaving about four hours after we started. For the first few hours, the abdominal cramping continued and finally stopped about ten hours after the chemo. Then I felt fine, thanks to those awesome steroids.

The next day I was back at the doctor's office for the Neulasta shot. This shot was designed to raise white blood cell counts during chemo. Depending on the chemo drug, this is a very common "part two" to the chemo infusion. My shot was administered roughly twenty-four hours after the infusion.

Bottom line: this was when the doctor recommended we change chemo regimens, because of the abdominal cramping. Don't be surprised if your world changes several times during chemo!

Unsolicited Advice

Start taking the offer of assistance!

Chapter 14

Action—Release Your Hair
(All about the Hair, Part Two)

Me: "I'm excited for you to visit this weekend."

Sister: "Me too! Anything I should bring?"

Me: "Hmm ... shampoo. I gave it all away when I lost my hair."

LOSING MY HAIR WAS very weird. It started with a "tingling" sensation at my scalp about two weeks after the first chemo infusion. My head was itchy and sensitive, but I couldn't stop touching it. Within only a day or two, the hair started to fall out much, much faster. One morning, I woke up to bald patches, and I'd had enough. I whacked it all off with a pair of clippers to a length about an eighth of an inch long.

The hardest part was showering for those first few days. It was outrageous how much hair could accumulate in the shower when it so short. My head was like a cue ball within about six days.

Shockingly, actually losing my hair was not traumatic. Cutting it short at the hair cutting party was much more emotional. I think this was because I started to associate losing my hair with being one step closer to kicking cancer's butt. Kicking cancer's butt was my ultimate goal anyway, so what was a little hair loss on the journey?

Okay—so that was the story of the hair on the top of my head, but we all have hair in other places too (ha-ha). One place I didn't mind losing hair was "down there." Yep—the "down there" hair also fell out. I would have thrown a party for this hair loss, but I couldn't figure out what to put on that cake. The "down there" hair fell out a week or two after the hair on the top of my head. For five glorious months, I had a perfectly kept Brazilian bikini wax.

I also lost the hair on my legs and much of the hair on my arms. Again, for five glorious months, I didn't have to shave! Talk about a silver lining to hair loss. Getting back into the routine of shaving was quite a drag.

I also lost a significant portion of my eyebrows and eyelashes. The oddest part of this hair loss wasn't the thinning I experienced during chemo, but the re-growth after chemo, which pushed out the rest of my eyebrows and eyelashes. I had 'baby' eyelashes for over a month. The eyelashes were there, but they weren't long enough for mascara. This made me mad, and my coworkers listened daily to the saga of my eyelashes.

Lastly, I lost my nose hair. Yes, you read that correctly, I lost my nose hair. I considered using nose hair in the title of this book. Talk about something unexpected; losing nose hair was bizarre, and nobody told me about it. As best I can tell, nose hair must help keep the snot in your nose. Because once I lost it, I had to keep a tissue close at all times. Otherwise, snot accidents happened, and little snot droplets would end up on paper, cards, and anything else I was looking at carefully! Talk about craziness. I ended up just as excited about my nose hair growing back as the hair on the top of my head.

Obviously, hair loss was good and bad. I chose to focus on the good and leave the bad for another day. I hope you can do the same.

Unsolicited Advice

Rejoice in the Brazilian bikini wax! Hair loss is good and bad. Try to focus on the fact you are one step closer to being cancer free!

Chapter 15

Action–Don't Forget to Laugh (Chemo Side Effect: Exhaustion)

Me: "I'm so tired."

Sister: "I'm sorry.

Me: "I get up in the morning and need a nap a couple of hours later."

Sister: "Napping is a good thing."

Me: "I guess. Okay, let's see if we can find a silver lining."

Sister: "Your kitty loves spending so much time sleeping next to you."

Me: "That's true. It's also forcing me to relax."

Sister: "That's a good thing."

Me: "Hmm ... that's all I can think of. I need a nap!"

A WORD ABOUT THE REST of the side effects ... *they sucked!* The next few chapters are dedicated to the myriad of fun and exciting side effects that graced me with their presence throughout chemotherapy. These chapters are not meant to scare you. These chapters are meant to give you a realistic view of the side effects and poke fun at the absurdity.

So first, let's talk about exhaustion. In addition to hair loss, this was an expected side effect for me. Basically, whether I wanted to or not,

I was forced into relaxing, sleeping, and generally doing nothing for a few days after the infusion.

My chemo sessions were on Thursdays, and by Saturday evening, the exhaustion kicked in. As more and more chemo sessions were in the rearview mirror, the exhaustion became worse due to cumulative effects. Basically, my body did not have a whole lot of time to recover between chemo sessions, and therefore, the exhaustion was worse each time.

Let's see if I can give you a description of my day to explain what I mean. As I said, I started to get really tired on Saturday evenings. I usually went to bed around nine or ten in the evening on Saturday. If I was lucky, I dragged myself out of bed by nine on Sunday morning. After a little tea and maybe reading the Sunday paper, I needed a nap. I usually curled up with my little kitty, and we napped on my bed or the couch until about one in the afternoon. I would then make a tremendous effort to eat something. I usually needed a nap again around four. After trying to eat something for dinner, I headed off to bed around eight. This cycle lasted Sunday and Monday, but by Tuesday, I could cut out the nap in the morning. By Wednesday, I usually didn't need a nap. I just went to bed around eight at night. I think you can now understand why I *loved* the steroids and looked forward to the three days around chemo when I wasn't exhausted.

To be honest, this side effect wasn't too terrible. Yes, I was tired, but sleeping for two days every fourteen was really manageable.

Unsolicited Advice

Take a break, and get some sleep! The medical oncologist advised me to take four days "off" from my life after the chemo. She was right!

Chapter 16

Action–Don't Forget to Laugh (Chemo Side Effects: Nausea, Inability to Taste, and Weight Gain)

Me: "I need a little sympathy."

Sister: "Okay. What's going on?"

Me: "I'm calling you from my bathroom floor."

Sister: "Ha-ha. I did that my entire pregnancy. Grab a pillow and make yourself comfortable."

Me: (laughing) "OMG! I'm so nauseous!"

Sister: (laughing) "Mute! Mute! The mute button is key to this conversation."

LOOKING BACK ON THE nausea and reading the descriptions I wrote in my blog, I can't help but laugh. Nausea sucked, but my sense of humor got me through it.

It felt like a train or a Mack truck had hit me. I missed the actual vehicle hitting me, as my bald head was stuck in the toilet for each round of nausea. Oh yeah—it happened …

It was kind of like the worst hangover ever with the added benefit of aches and pains (I'll get to the pain in another chapter). I was beckoned by my toilet often and couldn't resist the quality time we spent together. I even slept on my bathroom floor some nights because the cool tile felt great on my bald head. But don't worry; this only lasted for a couple rounds while I figured out how to use the nausea drugs. Here's the trick. You must start the nausea drugs at the first sign of nausea! If you wait, thinking it will pass or it's not too bad, you will spend the next three days trying to get ahead of the nausea. The nurses told me this, but I didn't understand. Once I figured this out, my toilet and I called a truce, and I was able to sleep again in my bed. Please, please, please take my advice and save yourself!

Let's talk about the inability to taste. I like food; therefore, changing taste buds and my inability to taste most foods was a real downer. My recommendation is to go buy some cancer cookbooks. I needed to experiment with spices, flavors, and temperatures. It was frustrating, and there were many times I would spend a significant amount of time cooking something and then summarily dismiss it after one taste.

For me, if a food had a smell, I was much more inclined to "taste" it. However, for others, any smells send them running for the toilet. You'll have to figure this one out for yourself. Some of the odd food choices that sustained me during chemo were chicken broth with roasted red curry paste, peas with blue cheese, and eggnog with almond milk. Yes, they were odd choices for sure.

Now is as good a time as any to talk about weight gain. I was under the impression that chemo patients lost weight, and given my love affair with nausea and my changed taste buds, I thought weight loss was a given. Boy, was I wrong! According to my friendly medical oncology nurses, between 60 and 70 percent of their patients gained weight. Yep—you read that correctly. Patients gained weight. As I started to pack on the pounds, I couldn't believe the indignity and absurdity of this craziness. I am sorry to report I gained eighteen pounds on chemo. It makes me freakin' angry just writing that sentence! I am now doing my damnedest to work off those pounds. Not much I could do about it during chemo—or maybe there was, but I was too tired to think about it. Whatever the case, don't be surprised if weight gain sneaks up on you and then hits you over the head. But stay strong and keep laughing. This too will pass, and as I pointed out earlier in this section, once I finished chemo, I felt as if I could take on anything. Those extra pounds don't stand a chance!

Unsolicited Advice

Get ahead of the nausea, and take the drugs at the first sign! Buy a couple of cancer cookbooks or find a few recipes online, and then experiment. Don't sweat the weight gain; concentrate on getting through chemo.

Chapter 17

Action—Don't Forget to Laugh (Chemo Side Effect: Chemically Induced Menopause)

Sister: "What are you doing?"

Me: "I'm sitting here with peas on my head."

Sister: (laughing) "You're what?"

Me: "I'm talking to you while balancing frozen peas on my head. It's hot flash hell in my house. Wait! The peas are melting. Let me go grab some frozen corn."

OH, THE DELICATE TOPIC of chemically induced menopause. If you are a man reading this book, feel free to skip this chapter.

I was forty-one years old when I was diagnosed with breast cancer. I did not expect to think about menopause (let alone write about menopause) for at least ten years. This damn cancer thing changed my life.

One of the anticipated side effects of chemotherapy was chemically induced menopause, which basically means I had all the fun and excitement of menopause (ceasing menstruation, hot flashes, mood swings, etc.) thrust upon me in a very short time frame. And if I am really "lucky" (written with extreme sarcasm ...), it's only temporary, and I will go through it again "naturally" later in life. Seriously—that's just wrong!

But that was the textbook version, not my version. I started menstruating pretty much nonstop once chemo started. And for all the women out there, not to be gross, but this was not "light," if you know what I mean, and I was not allowed to use tampons because of my increased risk for toxic shock syndrome (TSS) ... *You have got to be kidding me!* Talk about unfair; this was totally unfair. And you should have read "totally unfair" in a high school girl voice, because I felt like a high school girl. After about six weeks, I realized the bleeding might have been chemo related. Yes, it seriously took me six weeks.

I called my friendly nurses and gave them another crazy side effect to talk about. Exact quote—"Wow! Your hormones are whacked ..." Yes, yes they were! So what the heck did we do about it?

First, here's a little education. If you don't know (I didn't), during "that time of the month" your ovaries release a bunch of estrogen. (I don't know why, nor do I really care). With an estrogen-receptive cancer, it was apparently really bad to be flooding my body with estrogen continuously for six weeks. Who knew?

So, to counteract whatever my body was doing, I received a Lupron shot to shut down my ovaries and immediately send me into chemically induced menopause.

Hot flash hell started shortly after this shot. I experienced hot flashes all day long—hour after hour after hour after hour—and don't even get me started on the craziness all night long! The hot flashes started with a "warming" in my chest, followed by all-out sweating and the desire to shed every article of clothing and put my face in the freezer. The hot flashes only lasted a few minutes, but in those few minutes, I was on a warpath for ice and frozen peas for my bald head. Yep, I spent many days sitting at my computer with peas on my head.

To all my menopausal friends out there, I will never again laugh at hot flashes. Okay—well maybe I'll still laugh, but I'll be laughing with you.

Dawn Bontempo

Unsolicited Advice

Don't be surprised if your body does some crazy things. Frozen peas are an acceptable method of cooling a bald head.

Chapter 18

Action–Don't Forget to Laugh (Chemo Side Effects: Pain and Itching)

Me: "I feel as if little men are beating me with hammers."

Sister: "I can't say I know that feeling."

Me: "This pain thing feels like someone hammering on my bones from inside my body."

Sister: "Ouch!"

Me: "I know! These are evil little leprechauns!"

Sister: "I hope they bring you good luck though ..."

I AM SORRY TO SAY, the chemo pain was like nothing I had ever experienced. The friendly nurses said it was bone pain. As I told my sister in the above conversation, it felt like sharp hammering on my bones from inside my body. The pain rotated every minute or so, and I never knew where it would show up next. The pain itself was not excruciating, but it moved throughout my body with swiftness; my brain had a hard time wrapping itself around what the hell was happening.

I described bone pain as "little men beating me with hammers." For some reason, I pictured evil little men in mining carts traveling through my body, stopping only to hit me with little hammers. Maybe I watched too much *Snow White* or something. Let's see if I can describe the craziness: let's say the pain started with a sharp pain in my neck, followed by a pain in my toe, followed by a pain in my leg, followed by a pain in my arm, and then maybe back to my toe. It was the *weirdest* thing ... I took a lot of Vicodin.

Again, I should point out that for me, the pain was controlled with the Vicodin as long as I got in front of it. This is the same advice I gave for the nausea. Start taking the pain meds at the first sign of the pain. When I didn't, I spent days trying to get in front of it, much to my frustration and annoyance. By far, it was the mental gymnastics my brain engaged in when trying to understand the craziness that was the most frustrating.

In addition to the pain, I had the lovely experience of hives and itching. It all started with a slight itch on the back of my neck. I thought maybe the tag on my shirt was out to get me. So I ignored it. Within a couple of days, I was unable to ignore the itching and the hives, which had advanced down my back. I called my favorite nurses with yet another crazy, stupid side effect. The nurses advised taking Benadryl once every four to six hours to see if it cleared up.

So I took the Benadryl every four to six hours, and nothing happened. A week later, my entire back was covered in ugly, disgusting welts that had decided to travel to my arms and legs. *Nothing* (prednisone, Benadryl, Claritin, Allegra) was working, and I was ready to scratch myself with a wire brush until I bled! I finally had enough when the hives spread to my face. Feeling pretty sorry for myself, I dragged my hairless, hive-ridden, sarcastic self to the doctor's office once again.

This is when the next doctor was added to my speed dial. Off to the dermatologist I went. My sassiness was at an all-time high, and this was the closest I came to putting those Mardi Gras beads in my purse, but alas, I forgot them. Another powerful prescription, and I was as good as new in about three weeks. I also found out it wasn't hives, but a drug rash. Hey, here's a silver lining: without a cancer diagnosis, I would not know how prone I was to skin reactions from a variety of drugs.

Unsolicited Advice

Get ahead of the pain, and take the pain meds at the first sign! Expect the unexpected, and don't be thrown when your chemo journey takes a right turn.

Chapter 19

Action–Don't Forget to Laugh (Chemo Side Effect: Chemo Brain)

Me: "I live in a fog. I have chemo brain."

Sister: "That explains why you told me the same story three times yesterday."

Me: "I did?"

Sister: (laughing) "Yep, but I enjoyed it each time."

"CHEMO BRAIN" SHOULD BE the name of a very scary ride at Six Flags! I admit this was probably the side effect that I disliked the most. Yep—even more than the little men with hammers, the tasteless meals, or the exhaustion. Why did I dislike chemo brain so much? Because it was in my face every day!

Never heard of chemo brain? Let me enlighten you. I'll try to explain with my very personal definition.

1. I lived in a fog!

No, I didn't move to Washington State (ha-ha). I have an active imagination. Whereas for the bone pain, I imagined little men with hammers beating me, when I pictured chemo brain, I imagined myself walking disoriented down a foggy dirt road in the middle of nowhere.

Yep—I felt as if I were stumbling and disoriented on a foggy dirt road. In my imagination, I couldn't really see where I was going, but I knew I needed to be somewhere. I was also mad as hell! Let me give you an example. In one of my blogs, I used the word *cease*. I kid you not; I had to look it up in the dictionary! I could use it in a sentence; I even knew "cease fire" was a phrase … but my brain could not connect the dots, and I could not figure out if it meant "go" or "stop"! How scary is that? I started opening the dictionary on my computer *all the time*. Basically, tasks took me longer—both to comprehend and to process. I also found myself mixing up words—*patients* and *patience*, for example. I read and reread everything and hoped that I caught the mistakes. (Thanks to all who edited this book!)

2. I forgot everything!

I'm a list maker. I make lists for a lot of things. During chemo, I made lists for *everything*. I could stand up, take one step, and promptly forget the reason I stood up. And forget remembering the four things I needed at the grocery store. It was not going to happen. It was quite funny writing the blog associated with this chapter, as I kept forgetting what I intended to say.

The worst part was that I knew it was happening. I found myself trying like crazy to compensate. This was my new reality, and I hated it! I look back now and realize there were probably many times I repeated myself and told the same stories to the same people. My peeps were awesome. No one complained when I told the same stories again and again.

The forgetful fog disappeared about five or six months after chemo started. I was very happy to kick this side effect to the curb!

Unsolicited Advice

Not much you can do about chemo brain. Start making lists!

Chapter 20

Action–Don't Forget to Laugh
(Chemo Side Effect: Neuropathy)

Me: "I'm sending you a picture."

Sister: "A picture of what?"

Me: "I'm trying to capture the absurdity of a situation."

Sister: "Nice!"

Me: "I have frozen peas on my head and pink socks, a heating pad, and my cat on my feet."

Sister: (laughing) "Oh, definitely send me that picture!"

IN MY CASE, NEUROPATHY felt like my feet were soaking in ice water. There was pain, there was tingling, and there was stiffness. For the first week or two, I just thought my feet were exceedingly cold. Since I was also dealing with hot flashes, it was hysterical. I would have frozen peas on my head and colorful sock layers, a heating pad, and blankets on my feet. It made me laugh.

One night I made a startling discovery. My feet weren't actually cold. They were warm to the touch and only *felt* as if they were soaking in ice water. I didn't know about neuropathy, nor could I have anticipated my brain's interpretation, which forced an existence in which I needed to wear multiple layers of socks and a heating pad.

Good news—neuropathy was a normal side effect, and my friendly nurses were all over it. Once I explained my symptoms, I was given another prescription. The craziest part was the fact that it took me weeks to realize that my feet weren't cold and that this might be related to chemo. Keep watch for anything unexpected, and talk to the nurses. Learn something from me. Whatever it is, it's usually related to chemo.

Unsolicited Advice

Be aware of cold, tingling feet! This could be the first sign of neuropathy.

Chapter 21

Action—Don't Forget to Laugh
(Chemo Side Effects: Butt Abscess
and Other Frustrating Things)

Me: "I think I have to go to the urgent care."

Sister: "Why?"

Me: "There's an abscess on my ass, and it keeps getting bigger!"

Sister: (laughing). "A what? Are you kidding me?"

Me: "I'm a Victoria's Secret girl. My thong underwear is rubbing it."

Sister: "Why don't you just switch underwear so it doesn't rub?"

Me: "Never! Cancer can take my hair, but it will never take my underwear."

Sister: (laughing). "You are crazy! Go buy granny panty underwear."

Me: "Maybe some day. But first I'm off to urgent care. What a great way to spend a Friday night."

OH YES, THERE WAS a butt abscess! I think it started innocently enough as a blister. I bought a treadmill, and every morning I walked on it. After a couple of weeks, I could feel a blister near my butt crack. It got worse and worse as the weeks progressed. By the time it was the size of a nickel, it hurt enough to send me to urgent care.

After a mortifying appointment, which included me facedown on the exam table with my pants around my ankles while the doctor lanced, drained and took a sample for the lab, I was prescribed antibiotics. Lab results came back with a staph infection. Seriously, I couldn't catch a break.

I joked with my sister about the abscess on my ass, which was kind of lyrical but extremely painful and annoying. I didn't ask for pictures, and I didn't consider using *ass abscess* in the book title.

This was only the first instance where this Victoria's Secret girl was forced to reevaluate underwear choices. After this adventure, I was driven to buy "normal" underwear and wear them for a few months. Damn cancer!

The second underwear-shopping adventure was as a result of radiation. I was advised to only wear cotton bras with no underwire during radiation. This was to help with comfort when the skin started to become irritated. Ha! Cotton bras with no underwire were not easy to find for my size. The Victoria's Secret version stopped at a C cup. I ended up buying 100 percent cotton bras from Amazon.com. What did we do before Amazon.com?

Unsolicited Advice

Expect the unexpected, and laugh it off. I'm telling the world about thong underwear and an abscess on my ass; how bad can it be?

Chapter 22

Action–Try Something New (Acupuncture)

Me: "I was just stuck with something like twenty needles."
Sister: "Great!"
Me: "What? Great? Are you listening? I was just stuck with
   twenty needles!"
Sister: (laughing). "I'm guessing you just left acupuncture."
Me: "Yep! She made me stick out my tongue."
Sister: "Why?"
Me: "Apparently you can tell a lot from a person's tongue.
   Depending on the color and something else, she adjusts the
   needle positions."
Sister: "Wow. That's interesting."
Me: "I know. I think I'm hooked!"

I HAVE A NEEDLE PHOBIA. Therefore, paying someone to stick needles
in various places on my body and then "relaxing" for thirty to
forty minutes was quite a stretch. However, I *loved* acupuncture. If
you've never experienced it, let me walk you through a sixty-minute
appointment.

1. In the beginning, there was "discovery."

I began my appointments in a dimly lit room with soft piano music
playing. The acupuncturist, in a soothing and quiet voice, spent ten to

fifteen minutes asking me about my health since the last appointment. She focused on my chemo side effects and any other craziness my body was throwing at me. She finished the discovery phase by asking me to stick out my tongue. It always made me laugh! I once asked her what she's looking for on my tongue. I can't remember her exact answer (chemo brain!), but it was impressive. She also explained that she observed my nonverbal communication for clues into my "problem areas." I'm sure my sister could have told her a few "problem areas."

2. Next came the needles.

After determining the focus area for the session, I moved to a massage table with pillows at my head and my knees. This was when she stuck me with needles. It did not hurt. Well, okay, once in a while she hit something that made me realize she was poking me with needles, but 99.9 percent of the time, it did not hurt. I admit that during this phase, my eyes were shut, and I'm not sure a fire alarm would have made me open them. I really didn't want to see the needles.

3. Next, it was time to relax.

During the next phase, I was supposed to meditate. I was terrible at meditating. My mind was constantly thinking about something else like Mardi Gras beads. But I tried. I liked listening to the relaxing music, so maybe it was my own form of meditation.

4. Finally, the needles were removed.

The acupuncturist returned to the table about thirty minutes after I started meditating to remove those pesky needles. Then I was on my way.

Yeah, acupuncture!

Unsolicited Advice

Try something new! Acupuncture helped me tremendously!

Chapter 23

Action–Look on the Bright Side (Changing Chemo Drugs)

Sister: "Happy chemo day!"

Me: "Hey, thanks. I think I was high today."

Sister: (laughing) "Probably."

Me: "They gave me Benadryl via IV, and I felt like I was floating! I couldn't stop giggling. I could get used to that!"

Sister: (laughing) "What did the nurses say?"

Me: "They said my reaction wasn't normal, and they will probably decrease the dosage next time. It almost made the infusion fun! I was giggling and floating and generally very, very happy."

Sister: (laughing) "I never thought you'd say *infusion, giggling,* and *very, very happy* in the same conversation."

Me: "I know! Life is very good at the moment!"

FOR ME, ROUND FIVE of chemo was the start of the new drug Taxol. The infusion for this drug took forever. Let me walk you through it.

I arrived for my appointment at 9:00 a.m. (I previously arrived at 1:00 p.m.) After signing in, I chatted with everyone—yes, everyone—the ladies at the front desk, the billing department, the lab staff, and, of course, the nurses. I had to check in with the peeps!

At some point in the first fifteen minutes, one of the nurses cornered me and told me to pick a chair. I would finally decide on a chair around 9:15 a.m.

They stuck a needle into the port and then began administering the pre-treatment drugs. I received a steroid, Benadryl, an anti-nausea medication, and an anti-heartburn medication before the chemo drug. All of these were administered via IV.

My reaction to Benadryl was hysterical! I never had Benadryl via IV, but it was great. My mom accompanied me to the first session and watched firsthand the "high" I experienced. I told everyone I felt like I was lighter than air and able to fly out of the room; I also had a case of the giggles. It lasted a couple of hours the first time, but those blasted nurses cut my fun. They said I was too "high" the first time, so they cut my Benadryl dosage in half for the remainder of the sessions. Boo! Hiss! Boo! Hiss! I only felt as if I could fly for fifteen minutes for the last three sessions ... (big sigh).

In case you couldn't tell, I become hyper with Benadryl. Since I was receiving a good dosage at the infusion, I was ready to arrange a chemo party complete with dancing music. Unfortunately, the other chemo patients I normally chatted with slept after receiving Benadryl. So, while they slept, I bounced around in my seat.

After all the pre-treatment drugs, the nurses hooked up the Taxol, and for the next three and a half hours, I watched the IV *slowly* drip into my body. The whole process took about six hours.

Unsolicited Advice

Expect the unexpected, and laugh it off.

Chapter 24

*Action—Attend That
Support Group Meeting*

Sister: "Have you thought about going to a support group?"
Me: "Yep. But I haven't gone to a meeting."
Sister: "Why not?"
Me: "I don't know. I'm afraid of people with cancer."
Sister: "You can't catch it! You already have it!"
Me: (laughing) "Okay, but if the meeting sucks, I'm blaming
   you!"
Sister: (laughing) "Deal."

I ADMIT IT; I WASN'T sure a breast cancer support group was for me,
but several months after my diagnosis, I decided to give it a try. I
waited way too long!

The group I chose was the "young" women's breast cancer support
group. Score! A diagnosis at forty-one made me a "young woman," or
more specifically, it made me pre-menopausal. The hospital organizers
were brilliant in referring to us as young women. Even with my wrinkles
and saggy right breast, I wanted to be a young woman and associate
with young women!

It was my sister who finally convinced me to go. We (she) decided
I didn't have anything to lose—and we (she) gave me "permission"

to look at my phone if necessary and say, "Sorry—gotta go." Armed with my permission to leave, I attended my first meeting. I enjoyed the support group. Most of my new bald friends were just like me—a little overwhelmed but keeping their sense of humor.

This is one of those areas where I know I made a mistake. I should have attended a meeting right after I was diagnosed. I think I was scared of attending a sad, serious meeting and leaving feeling worse than when I walked in. This was *not* the case! It was empowering to be with women in various phases of treatment and discuss funny and frustrating things.

I also attended the American Cancer Society's "Look Good, Feel Better" class. It was awesome! I sat with five other cancer patients for two hours. We were given makeup instructions and a bag of makeup goodies. We also talked about wigs and scarves and hats. It was a fabulous class! I wish I had taken the class much, much earlier in my treatments.

Unsolicited Advice

Go to a support group meeting and find a "Look Good, Feel Better" class! It's fun to have bald friends!

Chapter 25

Action–Embrace the Emotional Hurricane

Me: "I am pissed off today!"

Sister: "Why?"

Me: "Because I have cancer!"

Sister: "You had cancer yesterday. What makes today different?"

Me: "I don't know. My hormones are whacked!"

Sister: "Hang in there! Remember, I'll always break you out of the loony bin!"

Me: (laughing) "Thanks! It's good to be able to count on an accomplice if I need one."

Sister: (laughing) "That's what family is for."

MY EMOTIONS WERE SO unpredictable during chemo. There were days when I was very happy. On those days, I walked around on cloud nine, feeling blessed to be alive and blessed with a positive attitude. I loved those days!

There were days when I was pissed off. I was really angry about the time the butt abscess showed up in my life. I was angry that I had cancer, angry that my body was falling apart, and angry that I couldn't sleep. That was a lot of anger!

There were days when I was sad and overwhelmed. Those were the days when I cried and curled up with my kitty. Those were also the days I needed my friends and family the most. They never disappointed me.

There were days when I was high on life! The last day of chemo was one of those days. I even did a "kickin' chemo to the curb" dance at the infusion center. The nurses and staff were fantastic. They laughed and hugged me through my dance.

I was blessed with a fantastic care team and supportive family and friends. All were inspiring and made me laugh throughout this journey. I want to thank them now for taking the time to be supportive. I could never have made it this far without them!

Unsolicited Advice

Roll with the emotions! And don't forget to say thank-you!

Part 4

Radiation

Me: "I'm drinking a lot more caffeine."

Sister: "Is radiation making you tired?"

Me: "Not tired like chemo, but scheduling radiation at 6:45 in the morning is exhausting."

Sister: "You could go in the afternoon, you know. You're making it more complicated."

Me: (silence) "Yep. But, there is a coffee machine at radiation. I just make a cup or two before heading off to work."

Sister: "Way to look at the positive."

Me: "Yep, and I'm caffeinated!"

RADIATION WAS NOT NEARLY as terrible for me as chemotherapy. The logistics were more challenging, but the side effects were very manageable. For me, radiation was Monday through Friday for thirty-four treatments, which meant seven weeks of fun. Everyone's experience will be different, but you can probably relax a little. Once radiation started, I had only a couple of more months before I declared victory!

Chapter 26

Action–Meet Even More Doctors and Learn Even More Vocabulary

Me: "I was tattooed today. I now have six tattoos!"

Sister: "What do they look like?"

Me: "They look a lot like freckles. I'm not sure you would notice them unless I pointed them out."

Sister: "Excellent."

Me: "I was hoping for butterfly!"

Sister: (laughing) "Maybe you can connect the dots someday."

ONCE CHEMOTHERAPY WAS COMPLETE, I graduated to a new doctor—a radiation oncologist. This was the doctor in charge of the radiation portion of my treatment. My initial meeting with the radiation oncologist lasted almost two hours, and she answered all my questions. She also laughed when I told her about breast cancer Mardi Gras and the beads. She was awesome!

She recommended thirty-four radiation treatments (yikes!) every day, Monday through Friday, starting approximately three weeks from my last chemo. Yes, this was seven weeks of fun and excitement.

To kick off radiation, I was scheduled for thirty minutes in a radiation simulator. What's a radiation simulator? Well, it is a machine that looks and functions just like the radiation machine, but it doesn't zap you with radiation. It is used to determine the best angle for zapping and to decide on the location for a patient's tattoos. Basically, I lounged while the doctor and the tech drew all over my breast in a purple sharpie and moved the machine around.

Did you read that? There were tattoos for radiation: six tattoos in my case! But much to my disappointment, the tattoos looked remarkably like freckles. I thought I'd get a good story, but instead I left with six dots and nothing resembling a butterfly.

When we finished the simulation adjustments, yet another digital camera emerged for photos of my left breast, which was now neatly marked with purple sharpie and tattoos. I couldn't help but giggle and picture purple sharpie Mardi Gras beads.

I also met with a new friendly nurse who went over side effects and skin care. There were two main side effects associated with radiation: skin reactions and fatigue.

Both of the side effects started for me about two to three weeks after beginning treatments. I'll talk specifically about them in another chapter.

Unsolicited Advice

Embrace the tattoos!

Chapter 27

Action–Try to Relax for Fifteen Minutes (Radiation Has Begun)

Me: "Radiation was really quick. The appointment was less than fifteen minutes."

Sister: "That's good, right?"

Me: "It is good. I pictured myself as the chalk outline in a murder mystery. I was lying on my back with my left arm in a sling above my head, and my feet were strapped together with a rubber band."

Sister: (laughing) "That doesn't sound like the chalk outline. It sounds like the actual victim."

Me: (laughing) "Hmm ... good point."

I CHOSE TO SCHEDULE RADIATION at 6:45 a.m. It's not for everyone, but I wanted my life to get back to normal. For me, that meant that I wanted to be in the office and working. By scheduling my zapping at 6:45 a.m., I was able to change into work clothes at the doctor's office and arrive at work around 7:30 a.m. It was perfect, even though it was complicated and exhausting to wake up at 5:45 a.m. every morning.

By this time, I was shockingly comfortable showing my boobs to strangers, and I began to imagine the craziest set of Mardi Gras beads to fit the situation. I'll get to that in a minute.

Each of the radiation appointments went something like this. First, I changed into a robe in a quaint dressing room equipped with small lockers. It was a nice spa feeling for about a minute and a half. Then the techs arrived and whisked me into the radiation room. I don't know what I expected, but the radiation machine looked like a giant X-ray machine, probably about eight feet tall. There was a robotic "arm" used to line up the machine with my tattoos. This "arm" and the machine rotated to ensure they shot the radiation at just the right angle.

In the radiation room, I took off my robe for even more strangers to see my boobs every morning and stated my name and birth date. I was then asked to lie down on a hard table face up with my head in a soft circle. My left arm was then placed in a sling above my head. As I told my sister in the dialogue above, I imagined I looked kind of like the chalk outline of a victim in a murder mystery. Then they strapped a giant rubber band around my feet to keep my feet still. I thought this was hysterical. The giant rubber band was not uncomfortable, and it did keep my feet still, but again, I point out, they strapped a rubber band around my feet.

The techs then positioned me and left the room. A loud noise and red lights startled me every morning. The noise lasted as long as the machine was zapping me. The techs then returned and positioned me again for the next zapping. This occurred three times before I was finished each morning. I didn't feel anything, but the noise was definitely startling each time the machine fired the radiation. The whole process lasted less than fifteen minutes.

In my head, the Mardi Gras beads for radiation were lightning bolts connected to a battery. I pictured the beads making loud noises and shooting rubber bands! How cool would that be?

The final eight radiation treatments were called "the boost." Whereas the first twenty-six sessions treated my entire breast and the lymph nodes, the final eight sessions treated just the area around the tumor removal site. There was more purple sharpie and drawing before we started "the boost." My particular artwork resembled an oval approximately four inches by two inches. The size of the area for the boost was too large for inconspicuous tattoos, so they used purple sharpie and a paint pen every day to make sure I was zapped in the right place.

In addition, the radiation machine was much closer to my body for "the boost." Check out the plate they install in the machine if you get a chance. It matched the purple sharpie mark on my boob. When I asked, they said each of the plates was specially cut for each patient. I thought this was pretty cool. I was lying on my side for "the boost," and there was no rubber band. Each of these treatments lasted only about five minutes.

I think I should have started radiation by giving the techs thirty-four sets of Mardi Gras beads. Each day when I left, they could have thrown me a set of beads! Why didn't I think of that sooner?

Unsolicited Advice

Relax! Looking back, I realize radiation wasn't too bad. Remember, you are one step closer to being done with all of this!

Chapter 28

Action–Don't Forget to Laugh (Radiation Side Effects)

Me: "I have a boob sunburn."
Sister: (laughing) "Envision yourself sunbathing at a clothing optional beach."
Me: (laughing) "Luckily, it's not too bad."
Sister: (laughing) "I'll take your word for it. No need to send a photo!"

APPROXIMATELY THREE WEEKS AFTER starting radiation, my side effects began. I referred to the most annoying side effect as the "boob burn." Yes, this side effect looked and felt like sunburn.

The skin was red, with raised dots similar to a rash in some places. Since we were also treating the lymph nodes, there was one particular red spot just above my collarbone. This spot sent me running to the doctor when I discovered the radiation was traveling through my body and making my back itch. I was freaked out! My imagination went into overdrive, and every morning, as the giant radiation machine pummeled my boob with invisible rays, I imagined myself starring in a science fiction film. In my sci-fi flick, cancer was the evil alien dictator (of course)! I was the heroine determined to beat the evil cancer in a battle across the galaxy. There was an old battle scar, a boob burn. The camera would zoom to my face as I grimaced and cursed the evil cancer! There were

Mardi Gras beads. The beads were the super secret, classified, guard-with–your-life weapon needed to destroy the evil cancer!

Whatever the evil cancer threw at me, I would defeat it! Let's take exhaustion, for example. I was tired, but it was nothing like chemo. I drank more caffeine and tried to go to bed at a reasonable hour. Take that, evil cancer!

Then my eyelashes and eyebrows fell out. I was annoyed, but I was a heroine now! Apparently because my eyelashes and eyebrows grew more slowly than the hair on my head, I was still losing them during radiation. I thought I was done with the hair loss crap after chemo! I was wrong, but I laughed in the face of cancer. Take that, evil cancer! Ha! Ha! Ha!

Then there were the toenails on my big toes. Early in chemo, the toenails on my both of my big toes turned black, but they never fell off. I was under the mistaken assumption that I had dodged losing my toenails. I was wrong. Toward the end of radiation, the toenails on my big toes popped off. Ugh! I cursed the evil cancer and vowed that next summer, I would have the prettiest toes in all the land. Take that, evil cancer!

The sci-fi movie in my head raged on. I even invented the coolest spaceship to transport me across the galaxy. The paint job resembled a Mardi Gras mask, and the interior included all the necessities of a heroine fighting evil cancer: a hair salon, a nail salon, and a super handsome masseuse. No matter what the evil cancer threw at me, I continued to kick its butt!

Even now, I laugh at the absurdity of my daily episode, but I kept giggling the entire seven weeks.

Unsolicited Advice

Radiation side effects are much, much better than chemo side effects! Invent your own story! Remember, you are one step closer to being done with all of this!

Chapter 29

Action—Get Out and Have Some Fun

Me: "I'm signing up for a bald photo shoot."

Sister: "Really?"

Me: "Yep. I found this site called *Shoots for a Cure*, where photographers donate their time for cancer survivors. I'm nervous about displaying my bald head, but whatever, I want to document this experience."

Sister: "I am so proud of you. You are out there taking back your life!"

DURING RADIATION, I STARTED to feel like a real person again. This prompted me to stop putting off activities and get out there for some fun.

Here's a crazy idea that I'm not sure I would have done before cancer. I was browsing Pinterest one day when I noticed a photo of a woman obviously going through cancer treatments. I clicked on the photo and was redirected to a site called *Shoots for a Cure*. It was awesome. Photographers donate a photo shoot for cancer survivors. Since I was interested in documenting my journey, I signed up. The photographer and I traveled to a local park for a photo session. I received the link to the proofs about a week later. Some were better than others. But, there were a few I will keep in a shoebox and take out when I need to remind myself of this journey and this fight. Get out there and do something new!

I also walked in the Race for the Cure. My sister traveled into town, and she and I along with a few friends walked a path around the monuments through the streets of DC. I was very proud in my pink survivor T-shirt. It was great to see all the breast cancer survivors and supporters. I intend to make this an annual event.

Unsolicited Advice

Take back your life! Get out there and do something you've never done or something that makes you happy.

Chapter 30

Action–Jump for Joy:
Hair Is Growing

Me: "My hair is gray!"

Sister: "So what? You can rock it now and color it in a couple of months."

Me: "You're so practical. My hair is gray!"

Sister: (laughing) "After all you've been through, what's a little gray hair?"

Me: (laughing) "Fine. But damn it, I'm mad that my hair is gray!"

Sister: "Let's focus on the positive. At least you have hair!"

The hair on the top of my head *finally* started to grow back during radiation. It was very soft and felt like peach fuzz, but like a bad dream, I couldn't tell if it was blond or gray! Gray! Gray! WTF! Gray! All of it! Gray! And when I complained about it to the young women's breast cancer support group, they all said their hair grew back gray. This was cruel and unusual punishment. However, within a couple of weeks, I started to see color other than gray. This was exciting! It was much more blond as it grew longer and longer.

I have no idea if this is an "old wives tale" or not, but I was told that the hair on my head would grow faster if it was able to breathe. So I ditched the hats, scarves, and headbands and started to rock the bald look. I told everyone "bald was the new blond."

And finally my nose hair started to grow back! I didn't really realize how much I would miss nose hair until it was gone. I am so thankful for the little things—even nose hair.

Unsolicited Advice

Rock the bald!

Part 5

Declaring Victory

Me: "I'm so excited to be done! No more chemo! No more radiation! Nothing. I'm done! Time to get back to my normal life."

Sister: "Ha! You think your life is *normal*?"

Me: "It is!"

Sister: "You're writing a book in your spare time. You're right—everyone does that."

Me: "Very funny. It feels good. I kicked cancer's butt! I'm a survivor!"

Sister: "And I couldn't be any more proud of you."

Surgery—done!
Chemotherapy—done!
Radiation—done!
Now what?

I WAS DAMN NERVOUS WHEN everything was done. I didn't see this cancer thing coming, but I sure wanted to see it leaving! I had been fighting for months, and then all of a sudden it was over. There was no graduation; there was no medal; there was nothing to mark this milestone. I wanted something or someone to tell me that I had won and that I had kicked cancer's butt! There was nothing ... not even doctor's appointments for over a month.

This was when I started to think of this journey as a marathon, partly for sanity and partly because it made sense. When someone finishes a marathon, she doesn't wait to be told that she won; she declares victory because she crossed the finish line!

I have heard fantastic finish line stories involving vacations, tattoos, reevaluating priorities, and skydiving. I can't understand the skydiving, but I certainly can get behind the other three ideas.

This book is my finish line. It marks the end of my Mardi Gras adventure, and I'm proud to say I'm a cancer survivor. It was not easy, but through it all I kept laughing. I wish the same for you!

About the Author

DAWN BONTEMPO IS A breast cancer survivor who is passionate about educating folks through humor. She is originally from Pennsylvania and currently resides in Arlington, Virginia. When she's not writing or fighting breast cancer, she can be found working as a civil servant who strives every day to make the world a little bit better.

About the Book

BREAST CANCER SURVIVOR DAWN Bontempo describes her journey in *Breast Cancer Mardi Gras: Surviving the Emotional Hurricane and Showing My Boobs to Strangers*. Her use of humor and sarcasm in a series of short action chapters will educate and delight the reader. This quick read is positive, optimistic, and funny.

Using conversations with her sister and her active imagination, Dawn chronicles her journey and provides unsolicited advice at the end of every chapter. From the initial "I have cancer" Facebook post to boob photos to the abscess on her butt, Dawn will keep you laughing as she educates you. She addresses tough topics during the diagnosis, surgery, chemotherapy, and radiation portions of her treatment. Using a style that makes you enjoy the absurdity of her life, she provides education, hope, and a good laugh.

CPSIA information can be obtained
at www.ICGtesting.com
Printed in the USA
FSHW012025230919
62308FS

9 781491 803158